THE COMPLETE LOW POTASSIUM DIET COOKBOOK

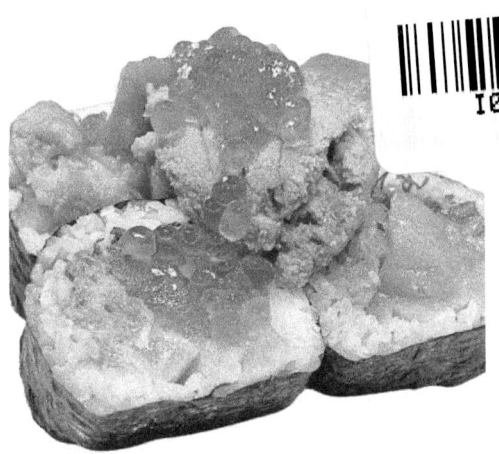

"30 Healthy Low Potassium Diet Recipes"

ALLIE NAGEL

Copyright © 2023 by Allie Nagel

DISCLAIMER

This cookbook is intended to provide general information and recipes.

The recipes provided in this cookbook are not intended to replace or be a substitute for medical advice from a physician.

The reader should consult a healthcare professional for any specific medical advice, diagnosis or treatment.

Any specific dietary advice provided in this cookbook is not intended to replace or be a substitute for medical advice from a physician.

The author is not responsible or liable for any adverse effects experienced by readers of this cookbook as a result of following the recipes or dietary advice provided.

The author makes no representations or warranties of any kind (express or implied) as to the accuracy, completeness, reliability or suitability of the recipes provided in this cookbook.

The author disclaims any and all liability for any damages arising out of the use or misuse of the recipes provided in this cookbook. The reader must also take care to ensure that the recipes provided in this cookbook are prepared and cooked safely.

The recipes provided in this cookbook are for informational purposes only and should not be used as a substitute for professional medical advice, diagnosis or treatment.

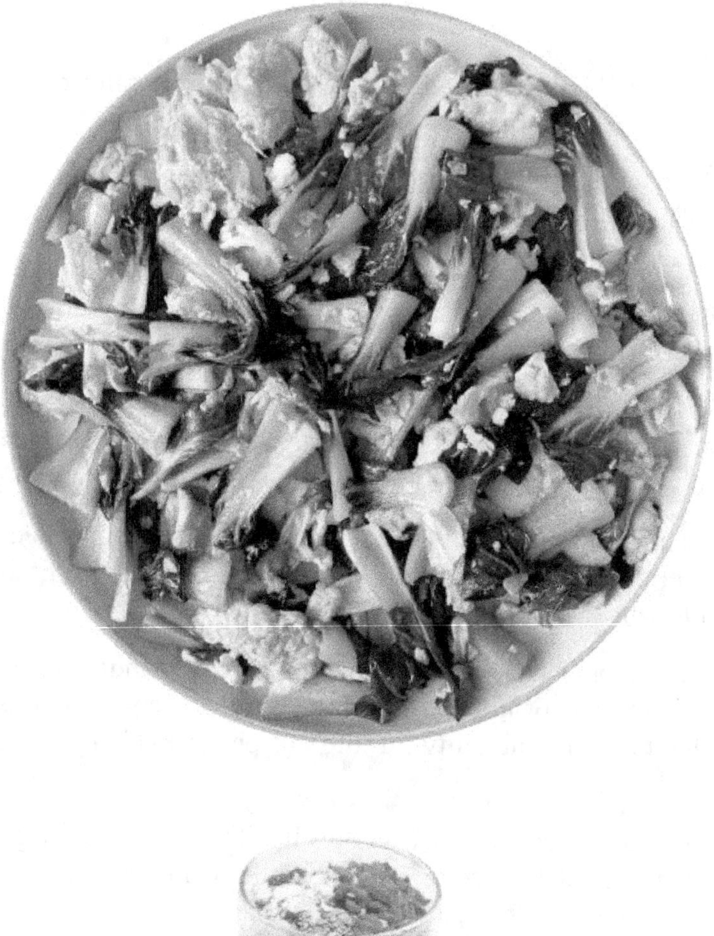

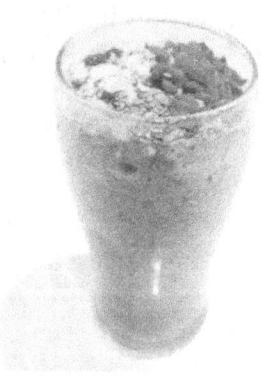

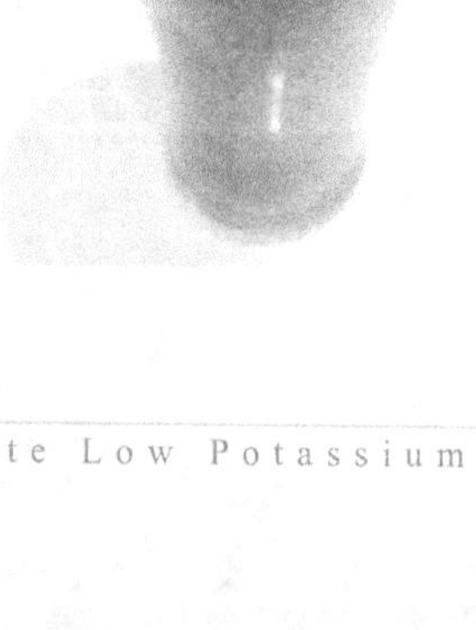

TABLE OF CONTENTS

INTRODUCTION

A low potassium diet is a nutritional approach aimed at restricting the intake of potassium, an essential mineral that plays a crucial role in various bodily functions, including muscle contractions, nerve impulses, and fluid balance.

While potassium is vital for maintaining proper physiological functioning, anyone with certain medical conditions, such as kidney problems or specific medications, may need to limit their potassium intake.

Foods rich in potassium include fruits like bananas, oranges, and melons, as well as vegetables such as spinach, potatoes, and tomatoes.

Dairy products, nuts, and certain meats also contribute to potassium levels. In a low potassium diet, you will typically reduce your consumption of these high-potassium foods to manage your potassium levels within a specific range.

Medical professionals often prescribe low potassium diets for conditions like chronic kidney disease, where impaired kidney function can lead to an accumulation of potassium in the blood.

Elevated potassium levels, known as hyperkalemia can result in serious health issues, including irregular heartbeats and muscle weakness.

Managing a low potassium diet involves careful food selection and portion control. It may also necessitate avoiding certain salt substitutes, which often contain potassium chloride.

Anyone on a low potassium diet should work closely with healthcare providers and dietitians to ensure they meet their nutritional needs while effectively managing their potassium intake.

Finally, a low potassium diet is a therapeutic dietary approach designed to control potassium levels, particularly for individuals with specific medical conditions.

It requires a conscientious effort to make informed food choices, emphasizing a balance between meeting nutritional needs and avoiding excessive potassium intake.

CHAPTER 1

BENEFITS OF A LOW POTASSIUM DIET

1. **Kidney Health:** A low potassium diet is often recommended for individuals with kidney problems, as it helps reduce the workload on the kidneys by minimizing potassium excretion.

2. **Heart Function:** Maintaining a balanced potassium level is crucial for heart health. A low potassium diet can be beneficial for those with heart conditions, as it helps regulate heart rhythm and prevent potential complications.

3. **Blood Pressure Control:** Reduced potassium intake can contribute to better blood pressure management, particularly in individuals sensitive to changes in potassium levels.

4. **Muscle Function:** By limiting potassium, a low potassium diet helps prevent excessive muscle contractions, spasms, and weakness, promoting optimal muscle function.

5. **Nerve Health:** Potassium is essential for nerve impulse transmission. A low potassium diet can be beneficial for individuals with nerve-related issues, ensuring proper nerve function without overstimulation.

6. **Fluid Balance:** Potassium plays a role in maintaining fluid balance in the body. A low potassium diet assists in managing fluid levels, which is crucial for individuals with conditions like edema.

7. **Reduced Hyperkalemia Risk:** For those prone to high blood potassium levels (hyperkalemia), a low potassium diet is a preventive measure to avoid potential complications associated with elevated potassium.

8. **Medication Interaction:** Some medications can elevate potassium levels. A low potassium diet helps mitigate the risk of adverse interactions between certain drugs and potassium-rich foods.

9. **Electrolyte Balance:** Balancing electrolytes, including potassium, is essential for overall health.

CHAPTER 2

TIPS AND TRICKS ON HOW TO FOLLOW A LOW POTASSIUM DIET

1. **Portion Control:** Manage portion sizes of high-potassium foods to keep overall potassium intake within recommended limits. Be mindful of serving sizes to avoid unintentional excess.

2. **Choose Low-Potassium Alternatives:** Opt. for low-potassium alternatives to commonly consumed high-potassium foods. For example, choose apples instead of bananas for a lower potassium fruit option.

3. **Cooking Techniques:** Certain cooking methods can reduce potassium content. Boiling and leaching vegetables in water can help lower their potassium content, making them more suitable for a low potassium diet.

4. **Limit High-Potassium Fruits:** While fruits are essential, choose fruits with lower potassium content, such as berries and apples, and moderate your intake of higher potassium options like oranges and bananas.

5. **Dairy Selection:** Choose lower potassium dairy options. For instance, opt for almond milk instead of cow's milk or limit cheese intake, as these can be high in potassium.

6. **Read Food Labels:** Pay attention to food labels to identify and avoid products high in potassium. This is crucial for processed and packaged foods, where hidden potassium sources may be present.

7. **Limit Salt Substitutes:** Many salt substitutes contain potassium chloride. Be cautious and choose alternatives without added potassium if you need to restrict your potassium intake.

8. **Meal Planning:** Plan meals in advance to ensure a balanced and low potassium diet. This can help you make intentional food choices and avoid last-minute high-potassium options.

9. **Educate Yourself:** Understand the potassium content of various foods to make informed decisions. Knowledge of potassium levels in common foods is key to successful adherence to a low potassium diet.

CHAPTER 3

14-DAY MEAL PLAN

DAY 1

Breakfast: Scrambled Eggs with Kale

Lunch: Grilled Chicken Salad

Dinner: Grilled Chicken Breast with Lemon Herb Marinade

DAY 2

Breakfast: Buckwheat Pancakes with Berries

Lunch: Turkey Wrap with Lettuce

Dinner: Baked Tuna with Herbed Olive Oil

DAY 3

Breakfast: Smoothie with Apple and Macadamia Milk

Lunch: Zucchini Noodles with Pesto

Dinner: Shredded Chicken with Vegetable Stir-Fry

DAY 4

Breakfast: Rice Cake with Peanut Butter

Lunch: Baked Tuna with Herbs

Dinner: Lemon Garlic Shrimp Skewers

DAY 5

Breakfast: Egg White Omelet

Lunch: Egg Salad Lettuce Wraps

Dinner: Baked Cod with Dill and Lemon

DAY 6

Breakfast: Apple and Berries Fruit Salad

Lunch: White Rice with Grilled Shrimp

Dinner: Cauliflower Rice with Grilled Vegetables

DAY 7

Breakfast: Low-Potassium Muffins

Lunch: Chicken and Vegetable Kebabs

Dinner: Broiled Turkey Burgers

DAY 8

Breakfast: French Toast made with White Bread

Lunch: Tofu and Broccoli Stir-Fry

Dinner: Spaghetti Squash Stir-Fry

DAY 9

Breakfast: White Rice and Cabbage Sauce

Lunch: Cauliflower Pizza with Chicken

Dinner: Garlic Grilled Shrimp Skewers

DAY 10

Breakfast: Omelet with Onions and Cottage Cheese

Lunch: Shredded Turkey Lettuce Cups

Dinner: Baked Chicken Wings with Herbs

DAY 11

Breakfast: Scrambled Eggs with Kale

Lunch: Grilled Chicken Salad

Dinner: Grilled Chicken Breast with Lemon Herb Marinade

DAY 12

Breakfast: Buckwheat Pancakes with Berries

Lunch: Turkey Wrap with Lettuce

Dinner: Baked Tuna with Herbed Olive Oil

DAY 13

Breakfast: Smoothie with Apple and Macadamia Milk

Lunch: Zucchini Noodles with Pesto

Dinner: Shredded Chicken with Vegetable Stir-Fry

DAY 14

Breakfast: Rice Cake with Peanut Butter

Lunch: Baked Tuna with Herbs

Dinner: Lemon Garlic Shrimp Skewers

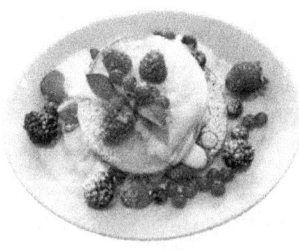

CHAPTER 3

NUTRITIOUS LOW POTASSIUM DIET RECIPES

BREAKFAST

Scrambled Eggs with Kale

Preparation Time: 10 Minutes

Serves: 4

Calories: 304 **Sugar:** 0g **Sodium:** 248mg

Ingredients:

4 large eggs

1 cup chopped kale (deveined)

Salt and pepper

1 tablespoon olive oil

Method of Preparation:

1. In a bowl, beat the eggs and season with salt and pepper.

2. Heat olive oil in a pan over medium heat.

3. Add chopped kale to the pan and sauté until wilted.

4. Pour the beaten eggs over the kale and stir continuously until the eggs are fully cooked.

5. Serve hot.

Buckwheat Pancakes with Berries

Preparation Time: 15 Minutes

Serves: 2

Calories: 150 **Sugar:** 1g **Sodium:** 200 mg

Ingredients:

1 cup buckwheat flour

1 tablespoon sugar (optional)

1 teaspoon baking powder

1/2 teaspoon salt

1 cup unsweetened almond milk

1 large egg

Cooking spray

Fresh berries for topping

Method of Preparation:

1. In a bowl, whisk together buckwheat flour, sugar (if using), baking powder, and salt.
2. In a separate bowl, beat the egg and mix it with almond milk.
3. Combine wet and dry ingredients and stir until just combined.
4. Heat a griddle or non-stick pan over medium heat and lightly coat with cooking spray.
5. Pour 1/4 cup of batter onto the griddle for each pancake.
6. Cook until bubbles form on the surface, then flip and cook the other side.
7. Top with fresh berries before serving.

Smoothie with Apple and Macadamia Milk

Preparation Time: 15 Minutes

Calories: 120 **Sugar:** 10g

Ingredients:

1 medium apple, peeled and chopped

1 cup unsweetened macadamia milk

1/2 banana (optional)

Ice cubes (optional)

Method of Preparation:

1. In a blender, combine chopped apple, macadamia milk, banana (if using), and ice cubes.
2. Blend until smooth.
3. Pour into a glass and serve immediately.

Rice Cake with Peanut Butter

Preparation Time: 5 minutes

Serves: 1

Calories: 150 **Sugar:** 2g **Sodium:** 70mg

Ingredients:

1 rice cake

2 tablespoons of low-potassium peanut butter

Method of Preparation:

1. Place the rice cake on a plate or a clean surface.
2. Stir the low-potassium peanut butter to ensure its well-mixed.
3. Spread the peanut butter evenly over the rice cake.
4. Optional: You can add a thin slice of a low-potassium fruit like banana or a sprinkle of cinnamon for extra flavor.

Egg White Omelet

Preparation Time: 15 minutes

Serve: 1

Calories: 120 **Sugar:** 2g **Sodium:** 200mg

Ingredients:

3 egg whites

1/4 cup diced bell peppers (choose low-potassium varieties)

1/4 cup diced onions

1/4 cup diced tomatoes (remove seeds to reduce potassium)

Salt and pepper

Method of Preparation:

1. In a bowl, whisk the egg whites until frothy.
2. Heat a non-stick skillet over medium heat.
3. Add the diced bell peppers, onions, and tomatoes to the skillet. Cook until softened.
4. Pour the whisked egg whites over the vegetables in the skillet.
5. Allow the eggs to set on the bottom, then gently lift the edges to let the uncooked eggs flow underneath.
6. Once the omelet is set, fold it in half with a spatula.
7. Season with salt and pepper.

Apple and Berries Fruit Salad

Preparation Time: 10 minutes

Serves: 1

Calories: 80 **Sugar:** 12g

Ingredients:

1 medium-sized apple, diced (choose a low-potassium variety)

1/2 cup strawberries, sliced

1/2 cup blueberries

1 tablespoon lemon juice

Method of Preparation:

1. In a bowl, combine the diced apple, sliced strawberries, and blueberries.
2. Drizzle the lemon juice over the fruits and toss gently to coat.
3. Refrigerate for a few minutes before serving for a refreshing taste.

Low-Potassium Muffins

Preparation Time: 30 Minutes

Serves: 2

Calories: 150 **Sugar:** 1g **Sodium:** 100mg

Ingredients:

1 cup all-purpose flour

1/2 cup oat flour

1/4 cup low-potassium baking powder

1/4 teaspoon salt

1/2 cup unsweetened applesauce

1/4 cup vegetable oil

1/2 cup sugar substitute (low-potassium)

2 large eggs

1 teaspoon vanilla extract

1/2 cup low-potassium fruits (e.g., blueberries)

Method of Preparation:

1. In a bowl, whisk together the all-purpose flour, oat flour, low-potassium baking powder, and salt.
2. In another bowl, mix together the applesauce, vegetable oil, sugar substitute, eggs, and vanilla extract.
3. Combine the wet and dry ingredients until just mixed. Fold in low-potassium fruits.
4. Spoon the batter into muffin cups lined with paper liners.
5. Place the muffin cups in the slow cooker. Cover and cook on low for 2-3 hours or until a toothpick inserted comes out clean.
6. Let the muffins cool before serving.

French Toast made with White Bread

Preparation Time: 25 Minutes

Serves: 2

Calories: 180 **Sugar:** 2g **Sodium:** 150mg

Ingredients:

4 slices low-potassium white bread

2 large eggs

1/2 cup low-potassium milk

1 teaspoon vanilla extract

1/4 teaspoon cinnamon

Cooking spray

Method of Preparation:

1. In a bowl, whisk together eggs, low-potassium milk, vanilla extract, and cinnamon.
2. Dip each slice of bread into the mixture, ensuring it's coated on both sides.

3. Heat a non-stick skillet or griddle and coat with cooking spray.

4. Cook each slice for 2-3 minutes on each side or until golden brown.

5. Serve with a sprinkle of powdered sugar or a drizzle of low-potassium syrup.

White Rice and Cabbage Sauce

Preparation Time: 50 Minutes

Serves:

Calories: 200 **Sugar:** 3g **Sodium:** 300mg

Ingredients:

1 cup white rice

2 cups shredded cabbage

1 can (14 oz) low-potassium diced tomatoes

1 teaspoon garlic powder

1 teaspoon onion powder

Salt and pepper

2 cups low-potassium vegetable broth

Method of Preparation:

1. In the slow cooker, combine rice, shredded cabbage, diced tomatoes, garlic powder, onion powder, salt, and pepper.
2. Pour the vegetable broth over the ingredients and stir.
3. Cover and cook on low for 3-4 hours or until the rice is tender.
4. Adjust seasoning if needed before serving.

Omelet with Onions and Cottage Cheese

Preparation Time: 15 Minutes

Serves: 2

Calories: 180 **Sugar:** 2g **Sodium:** 200mg

Ingredients:

2 large eggs

1/4 cup low-potassium cottage cheese

1/4 cup chopped onions

Salt and pepper

1 teaspoon olive oil (for greasing)

Method of Preparation:

1. In a bowl, beat the eggs and mix in the cottage cheese, chopped onions, salt, and pepper.
2. Heat the olive oil in a skillet over medium heat.
3. Pour the egg mixture into the skillet and cook until the edges set.
4. Lift the edges to let uncooked eggs flow underneath.
5. When the omelet is mostly set, fold it in half and cook until the eggs are fully cooked.
6. Serve warm.

LUNCH

Grilled Chicken Salad

Preparation Time: 25 minutes

Serves: 4

Calories: 250 **Sugar:** 6g **Sodium:** 300mg

Ingredients:

1 lb. boneless, skinless chicken breasts

6 cups mixed salad greens (lettuce, spinach, arugula, etc.)

1 cup cherry tomatoes, halved

1 cucumber, sliced

1/2 red onion, thinly sliced

1/4 cup balsamic vinaigrette dressing (low-potassium version)

Salt and pepper

Olive oil for grilling

Method of Preparation:

1. Season the chicken breasts with salt and pepper.
2. Heat a grill or grill pan over medium-high heat and lightly brush with olive oil.
3. Grill the chicken for 6-8 minutes per side or until fully cooked.
4. Let the chicken rest for a few minutes before slicing it into thin strips.
5. In a large bowl, combine the salad greens, cherry tomatoes, cucumber, and red onion.
6. Add the sliced grilled chicken on top.
7. Drizzle the balsamic vinaigrette dressing over the salad.

8. Toss everything gently to combine.

9. Serve immediately.

Turkey Wrap with Lettuce

Preparation Time: 15 minutes

Serves: 4

Calories: 180 **Sugar:** 2g **Sodium:** 250mg

Ingredients:

8 large lettuce leaves (use iceberg or romaine)

1 lb. turkey breast, thinly sliced

1 cup shredded carrots

1/2 cup hummus (low-potassium version)

1/4 cup chopped fresh parsley

Salt and pepper

Method of Preparation:

1. Lay out the lettuce leaves on a clean surface.

2. Spread a thin layer of hummus on each lettuce leaf.

3. Place a few slices of turkey on each leaf.

4. Sprinkle shredded carrots and chopped parsley on top.

5. Season with salt and pepper.

6. Roll the lettuce leaves, securing them with toothpicks if needed.

7. Serve immediately.

Zucchini Noodles with Pesto

Preparation Time: 20 minutes

Serves: 4

Calorie: 220 **Sugar:** 3g **Sodium:** 150mg

Ingredients:

4 medium zucchinis, spiralized into noodles

1 cup cherry tomatoes, halved

1/2 cup homemade basil pesto (low-potassium version)

1/4 cup pine nuts, toasted

Salt and pepper

Method of Preparation:

1. Spiralize the zucchinis into noodles.

2. In a large pan, sauté the zucchini noodles over medium heat for 2-3 minutes until just tender.

3. Add the cherry tomatoes and cook for an additional 1-2 minutes.

4. Stir in the basil pesto and toss until everything is well coated.

5. Season with salt and pepper.

6. Transfer to a serving dish and sprinkle toasted pine nuts on top.

7. Serve immediately.

Baked Tuna with Herbs

Preparation Time: 10 minutes

Serves: 2

Calories: 200 **Sugar:** 0g **Sodium:** 200

Ingredients:

2 cans of low-sodium tuna, drained

1 tablespoon of olive oil

1 teaspoon of dried oregano

1 teaspoon of dried thyme

1 teaspoon of lemon juice

Salt and pepper

Method of Preparation:

1. Preheat your oven to 375°F (190°C).
2. In a bowl, mix the drained tuna with olive oil, oregano, thyme, lemon juice, salt, and pepper.
3. Place the tuna mixture in a baking dish.
4. Bake for 15-20 minutes or until the top is golden brown.
5. Serve warm.

Egg Salad Lettuce Wraps

Ingredients:

4 hard-boiled eggs, chopped

1/4 cup mayonnaise (low-fat or egg-free, if needed)

1 teaspoon mustard

2 tablespoons finely chopped celery

Salt and pepper

Iceberg lettuce leaves for wrapping

Method of Preparation:

1. In a bowl, mix the chopped eggs, mayonnaise, mustard, celery, salt, and pepper.
2. Spoon the egg salad onto individual iceberg lettuce leaves.
3. Wrap the lettuce around the egg salad, creating lettuce wraps.
4. Serve chilled.

Preparation Time: 15 minutes

Serves: 2

Calories: 180 **Sugar:** 1g **Sodium:**

White Rice with Grilled Shrimp

Preparation Time: 30 minutes

Serves: 2

Calories: 300 **Sugar:** 0g **Sodium:** 250mg

Ingredients:

1 cup white rice, uncooked

1 pound of shrimp, peeled and deveined

1 tablespoon olive oil

1 teaspoon garlic powder

1 teaspoon onion powder

Salt and pepper

Fresh parsley for garnish (optional)

Method of Preparation:

1. Cook the white rice according to the package instructions.
2. In a bowl, toss the shrimp with olive oil, garlic powder, onion powder, salt, and pepper.
3. Grill the shrimp until they are opaque and cooked through.
4. Serve the grilled shrimp over the cooked white rice.
5. Garnish with fresh parsley if desired.

Chicken and Vegetable Kebabs

Preparation Time: 15 minutes

Serves: 4

Calories: 250 **Sugar:** 4g **Sodium:** 120mg

Ingredients:

1-pound boneless, skinless chicken breasts, cut into cubes

1 zucchini, sliced

1 bell pepper, sliced

1 red onion, sliced

1 cup cherry tomatoes

2 tablespoons olive oil

2 cloves garlic, minced

1 teaspoon dried oregano

Salt and pepper

Method of Preparation:

1. In a bowl, mix olive oil, minced garlic, dried oregano, salt, and pepper.
2. Thread chicken, zucchini, bell pepper, red onion, and cherry tomatoes onto skewers.
3. Place the skewers in the slow cooker.
4. Pour the olive oil mixture over the skewers.

5. Cook on low for 4-6 hours or until the chicken is cooked through.

6. Serve with a side of renal-friendly grain like quinoa or brown rice.

Tofu and Broccoli Stir-Fry

Preparation Time: 15 minutes

Serves: 4

Calories: 220 **Sugar:** 3g **Sodium:** 300mg

Ingredients:

1 block firm tofu, pressed and cubed

4 cups broccoli florets

1 carrot, julienned

2 tablespoons low-sodium soy sauce

1 tablespoon rice vinegar

1 tablespoon sesame oil

1 tablespoon ginger, minced

2 cloves garlic, minced

1 teaspoon cornstarch

Sesame seeds for garnish (optional)

Method of Preparation:

1. In a bowl, mix soy sauce, rice vinegar, sesame oil, minced ginger, minced garlic, and cornstarch.
2. Place tofu, broccoli, and julienned carrot in the slow cooker.
3. Pour the sauce over the ingredients.
4. Gently stir to coat the tofu and vegetables with the sauce.
5. Cook on low for 3-4 hours.
6. Serve over renal-friendly grains like quinoa or brown rice, garnished with sesame seeds if desired.

Cauliflower Pizza with Chicken

Preparation Time: 20 minutes

Serves: 6

Calories: 180 **Sugar:** 5g **Sodium:** 220mg

Ingredients:

1 medium cauliflower, grated

2 cups cooked chicken, shredded

1 cup low-sodium tomato sauce

1 teaspoon dried oregano

1 teaspoon dried basil

1/2 teaspoon garlic powder

1 cup low-fat mozzarella cheese, shredded

Your favorite pizza toppings (e.g., bell peppers, olives)

Method of Preparation:

1. In a bowl, combine grated cauliflower, shredded chicken, tomato sauce, oregano, basil, and garlic powder.

2. Transfer the mixture to the slow cooker and spread it evenly.

3. Cook on low for 2-3 hours or until the cauliflower is tender.

4. Sprinkle shredded mozzarella cheese over the cauliflower mixture.

5. Cover and cook for an additional 30 minutes or until the cheese is melted.

6. Add your favorite pizza toppings.

7. Serve warm.

Shredded Turkey Lettuce Cups

Preparation Time: 15 minutes

Serves: 4

Calories: 180 **Sugar:** 2g **Sodium:** 200mg

Ingredients:

1-pound boneless, skinless turkey breast

1 cup low-sodium chicken broth

1 tablespoon low-sodium soy sauce

1 tablespoon rice vinegar

1 tablespoon ginger, minced

2 cloves garlic, minced

1 teaspoon sesame oil

1/2 cup water chestnuts, chopped

1/4 cup green onions, chopped

1 head iceberg lettuce, leaves separated

Method of Preparation:

1. Place turkey breast in the slow cooker.
2. In a bowl, mix chicken broth, soy sauce, rice vinegar, minced ginger, minced garlic, and sesame oil.
3. Pour the mixture over the turkey.
4. Cook on low for 5-7 hours or until the turkey is tender and easily shredded.
5. Shred the turkey using forks.
6. Stir in water chestnuts and green onions.
7. Serve the shredded turkey mixture in lettuce cups.

DINNER

Grilled Chicken Breast with Lemon Herb Marinade

Preparation Time: 10 minutes

Serves: 4

Calories: 200 **Sodium:** 500mg

Ingredients:

4 boneless, skinless chicken breasts

1/4 cup olive oil

2 tablespoons lemon juice

1 teaspoon dried oregano

1 teaspoon dried thyme

1 teaspoon dried rosemary

Salt and pepper

Method of Preparation:

1. In a small bowl, mix together olive oil, lemon juice, dried oregano, dried thyme, dried rosemary, salt, and pepper to create the marinade.
2. Place chicken breasts in the slow cooker.
3. Pour the marinade over the chicken, ensuring each piece is well-coated.
4. Cook on low for 4-6 hours or until the chicken is cooked through and tender.
5. Serve the grilled chicken breasts with your favorite renal-friendly sides.

Baked Tuna with Herbed Olive Oil

Preparation Time: 10 minutes

Serves: 4

Calories: 250 **Sodium:** 50mg

Ingredients:

4 tuna steaks

1/4 cup olive oil

2 tablespoons chopped fresh parsley

1 tablespoon chopped fresh basil

1 tablespoon chopped fresh dill

Salt and pepper

Lemon wedges for serving

Method of Preparation:

1. Place tuna steaks in the slow cooker.
2. In a small bowl, mix together olive oil, chopped parsley, chopped basil, chopped dill, salt, and pepper to create the herbed olive oil mixture.

3. Pour the herbed olive oil mixture over the tuna steaks.

4. Cook on low for 2-3 hours or until the tuna is cooked to your liking.

5. Serve the baked tuna steaks with lemon wedges and renal-friendly sides.

Shredded Chicken with Vegetable Stir-Fry

Preparation Time: 15 minutes

Serves: 4

Calories: 220 **Sodium:** 200

Ingredients:

4 boneless, skinless chicken breasts

2 cups mixed vegetables (broccoli, bell peppers, carrots), chopped

1/4 cup low-sodium soy sauce

2 tablespoons olive oil

1 tablespoon minced garlic

1 tablespoon minced ginger

Salt and pepper

Method of Preparation:

1. Place chicken breasts in the slow cooker.
2. In a small bowl, mix together soy sauce, olive oil, minced garlic, minced ginger, salt, and pepper.
3. Pour the sauce over the chicken.
4. Cook on low for 4-6 hours or until the chicken is easily shredded with a fork.
5. Shred the chicken and mix it with the cooked vegetables in a separate pan or wok for a stir-fry.
6. Serve the shredded chicken and vegetable stir-fry with renal-friendly sides.

Lemon Garlic Shrimp Skewers

Preparation Time: 20 Minutes

Serves: 2

Calories: 150 **Sugar:** 0g **Sodium:** 200mg

Ingredients:

1 pound shrimp, peeled and deveined

2 tablespoons olive oil

2 tablespoons fresh lemon juice

3 cloves garlic, minced

1 teaspoon dried oregano

1 teaspoon dried thyme

Salt and pepper

Lemon wedges for serving

Method of Preparation:

1. In a bowl, mix olive oil, lemon juice, minced garlic, oregano, thyme, salt, and pepper to create the marinade.
2. Add shrimp to the marinade, ensuring they are well-coated. Let it marinate for at least 30 minutes.
3. Thread shrimp onto skewers.
4. Place the skewers in the slow cooker.
5. Cook on low for 1-2 hours until shrimp are opaque and cooked through.
6. Serve with lemon wedges.

Baked Cod with Dill and Lemon

Preparation Time: 25 Minutes

Serves: 1

Calories: 180 **Sugar:** 0g **Sodium:** 150mg

Ingredients:

4 cod fillets

2 tablespoons olive oil

2 tablespoons fresh lemon juice

2 cloves garlic, minced

1 tablespoon fresh dill, chopped

Salt and pepper

Lemon slices for garnish

Method of Preparation:

1. Preheat the slow cooker on low.
2. In a bowl, mix olive oil, lemon juice, minced garlic, chopped dill, salt, and pepper to create the marinade.
3. Place cod fillets in the slow cooker.

4. Pour the marinade over the cod fillets.

5. Cook on low for 2-3 hours until the cod is flaky and cooked through.

6. Garnish with lemon slices before serving.

Cauliflower Rice with Grilled Vegetables

Preparation Time: 30 Minutes

Serves: 2

Calories: 120 **Sugar:** 6g **Sodium:** 100mg

Ingredients:

1 head cauliflower, grated to resemble rice

1 zucchini, sliced

1 bell pepper, sliced

1 cup cherry tomatoes, halved

2 tablespoons olive oil

1 teaspoon dried Italian herb

Salt and pepper

Fresh parsley for garnish

Method of Preparation:

1. In a bowl, toss cauliflower rice, sliced zucchini, bell pepper, and cherry tomatoes with olive oil, dried Italian herbs, salt, and pepper.
2. Transfer the mixture to the slow cooker.
3. Cook on low for 2-3 hours until vegetables are tender.
4. Garnish with fresh parsley before serving.

Broiled Turkey Burgers

Preparation Time: 15 minutes

Serves: 4

Calories: 250 **Sugar: Sodium:**

Ingredients:

1 pound ground turkey (lean)

1/4 cup finely chopped onion

1/4 cup chopped fresh parsley

1 teaspoon garlic powder

1 teaspoon onion powder

Salt and pepper

Whole wheat burger buns

Lettuce, tomato, and other preferred toppings

Method of Preparation:

1. In a mixing bowl, combine ground turkey, chopped onion, parsley, garlic powder, onion powder, salt, and pepper. Mix well.
2. Shape the mixture into burger patties.
3. Preheat the broiler.
4. Broil the turkey burgers for about 5-7 minutes per side or until they reach an internal temperature of 165°F (74°C).
5. Toast the whole wheat burger buns.
6. Serve the turkey burgers on the buns, topped with lettuce, tomato, and other preferred toppings.

Spaghetti Squash Stir-Fry

Preparation Time: 20 minutes

Serves: 4

Calories: 300 **Sugar:** 3g **Sodium:** 100mg

Ingredients:

1 medium-sized spaghetti squash

1 pound chicken breast, diced

2 cups broccoli florets

1 bell pepper, thinly sliced

1 carrot, julienned

2 tablespoons low-sodium soy sauce

1 tablespoon olive oil

1 teaspoon minced garlic

1 teaspoon minced ginger

Salt and pepper

Green onions for garnish

Method of Preparation:

1. Cut the spaghetti squash in half lengthwise and remove the seeds.
2. Place the squash halves in the slow cooker.

3. In a separate bowl, combine chicken, broccoli, bell pepper, carrot, soy sauce, olive oil, garlic, ginger, salt, and pepper. Mix well.
4. Add the chicken and vegetable mixture to the slow cooker, placing it around the spaghetti squash.
5. Cook on low for 4-6 hours or until the chicken is cooked through and the squash is tender.
6. Using a fork, shred the spaghetti squash into "noodles."
7. Serve the stir-fry over the spaghetti squash noodles, garnished with green onions.

Garlic Grilled Shrimp Skewers

Preparation Time: 15 minutes

Serves: 4

Calories: 150 **Sodium:** 120mg

Ingredients:

1-pound large shrimp, peeled and deveined

2 tablespoons olive oil

3 cloves garlic, minced

1 teaspoon paprika

1 teaspoon dried oregano

Salt and pepper

Lemon wedges for serving

Method of Preparation:

1. In a bowl, mix shrimp with olive oil, minced garlic, paprika, oregano, salt, and pepper.
2. Thread the shrimp onto skewers.
3. Preheat the slow cooker to low.
4. Place the skewers in the slow cooker and cook for 30-40 minutes or until the shrimp are opaque and cooked through.
5. Serve the shrimp skewers with lemon wedges.

Baked Chicken Wings with Herbs

Preparation Time: 15 minutes

Serves: 4

Calories: 200 **Sodium:** 200mg

Ingredients:

2 pounds chicken wings, split at joints, tips discarded

2 tablespoons olive oil

1 teaspoon dried thyme

1 teaspoon dried rosemary

1 teaspoon dried oregano

1 teaspoon garlic powder

Salt and pepper

Fresh parsley for garnish (optional)

Method of Preparation:

1. Preheat the slow cooker to low.
2. In a bowl, toss chicken wings with olive oil, thyme, rosemary, oregano, garlic powder, salt, and pepper.
3. Place the seasoned wings in the slow cooker.
4. Cook on low for 4-6 hours or until the wings are cooked through and crispy.
5. Optionally, broil the wings for a few minutes to achieve extra crispiness.
6. Garnish with fresh parsley if desired.

CONCLUSION

In conclusion, this book serves as a valuable resource for you seeking to manage your potassium intake while still enjoying delicious and nutritious meals.

By carefully selecting and combining ingredients, I've crafted a collection of recipes that not only adhere to low potassium guidelines but also prioritize flavor, variety, and overall well-being.

I understand the challenges that come with dietary restrictions, and my goal is to provide a practical and enjoyable solution for you to navigate a low potassium lifestyle.

Through these recipes, I aim to empower you to make informed choices that support your health without compromising on taste.

Whether you're exploring new flavors or adapting familiar recipes, this cookbook encourages creativity in the kitchen while maintaining a focus on renal-friendly ingredients.

Remember, maintaining a balanced and nutritious diet is a crucial aspect of overall health, and I hope this cookbook makes that journey more accessible and enjoyable.

As always, it is advisable to consult with healthcare professionals or registered dietitians for personalized dietary advice, especially for those with specific medical conditions.

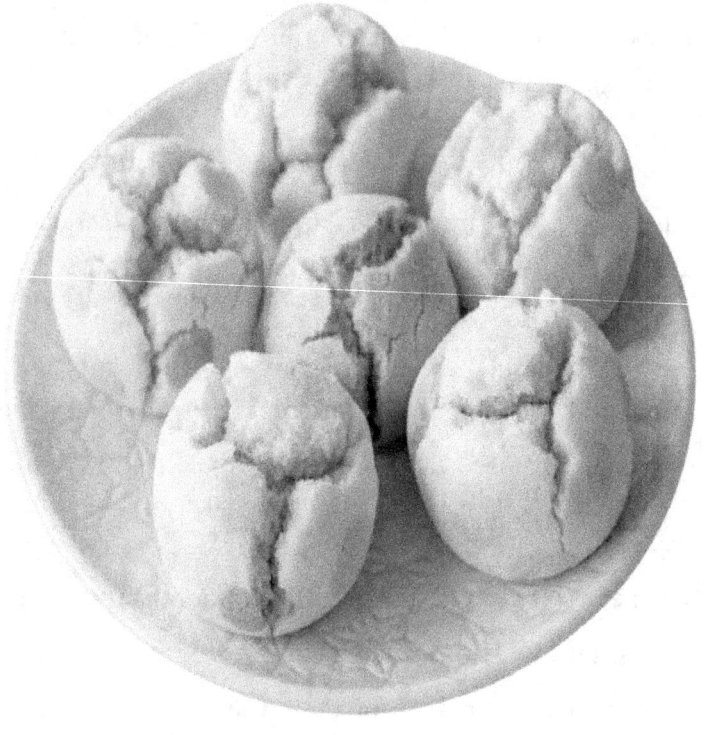